ESPECIALLY FOR WOMEN

Achieve Hormonal Balance Naturally

YOUR BODY · YOUR CHOICE

Natural Treatments for PMS, Menopause,
Osteoporosis & Breast Health

BY

Dr. Angela Stengler *&* Dr. Mark Stengler

FACTOR R&D TECHNOLOGIES LTD.

Copyright © 2000 Angela Stengler

Illustrations: Ernie Thomsen
Photography: Kent Kallberg
Design: Stephen Rank
Editor: Eunice Kortegaard

For information contact:
Factor R&D Technologies Ltd.,
Suite 308
10 Sierra Morena Mews S.W.,
Calgary, AB., Canada
T3H 3K5

ISBN 0-9687158-0-X

First printing April 2000

Printed in Canada

"Being a woman is not a disease!"

Dr. Angela Stengler

This book is dedicated to women who are seeking natural ways to enhance their health and happiness throughout their lives.

CONTENTS

A word about the authors

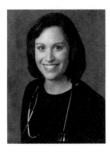

Dr. Angela Stengler, ND, HHP , is a popular and respected naturopathic doctor. Her expertise in women and children's health makes her a frequent guest of radio and television programs. She received her Bachelor's degree from Pitzer College, and her four-year Doctorate of Naturopathic Medicine, with extra training in obstetrics and pediatrics, from the National College of Naturopathic Medicine in Portland, Oregon. She is also co-author of *Menopause Relief, Build Strong Bones, Natural Solutions for PMS,* and *Your Child's Health.* Dr. Angela and her husband Mark host a weekly natural medicine radio show *The Natural Physician*™ aired throughout southern California, and across the world via the Internet.

Angela and Mark are sought-after speakers on many natural health subjects and and their latest book, *Your Vital Child* is being hailed as the world's leading reference children's natural healthcare. *Your Vital Child* will be published by Rodale Press.

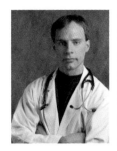 **Dr. Mark Stengler,** ND, CHT, HHP, a renowned licensed naturopathic doctor, author, and lecturer, has helped thousands on the road to better health. Dr. Stengler completed his pre-medical studies at the University of Calgary, and received his four-year doctorate of naturopathic medicine degree and certification in homeopathy from the National College of Naturopathic Medicine in Portland, Oregon. Currently, he is practising in La Jolla, California and is an associate Clinical Professor at the National College of Naturopathic Medicine in Portland, Oregon. Dr. Stengler was trained as a general family practitioner specializing in natural healthcare including nutrition, supplements, herbal therapy, homeopathy, and he is completing his master's degree in acupuncture and Oriental medicine. Dr. Stengler is also a consultant to the health food industry and author of a Canadian best seller, *The Natural Physician: Your Guide for Common Ailments* and other books and publications. Dr. Stengler is co-host, with Angela, of *The Natural Physician*™ radio program and he serves on the medical advisory board for Rodale Press.

Introduction

S ociety would have us believe that being a woman is a disease, and any symptoms signal just another unpleasant phase of womanhood best suppressed with powerful drugs, no matter what their side effects. As women we sometimes tend to agree, especially if it's around that time of the month. We want to eat everything in sight, we're bloated, weepy and cranky, or we're trying to keep our composure around family and friends while we're experiencing another fiery hot flash.

That's why I'm writing this book. First, to tell you that it's not a disease to be a woman. Knowing what's happening to our body is central to living full, rich lives. Second, there are natural ways to manage the hormones that pull and tug at us at every stage of our lives. We hope that the suggestions in this book will help you to understand the natural feminine rhythms that make us unique and calm the hormonal storms that can give us so much discomfort. The healthful strategies suggested will help you from puberty to menopause and beyond.

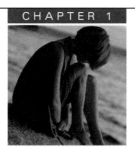

CHAPTER 1

PMS – It's real, but it can be managed

Some women dread the two weeks before their period. They just wish the bleeding would start so their symptoms would end. In my practice I treat premenstrual syndrome (PMS). I have experienced PMS, and I have friends and family who suffer from PMS. These symptoms are not a figment of the imagination. They are real symptoms and women need real relief. Some women cannot even function during this time.

As you read this book, consider the treatment options to ease PMS. Some of you may find relief by simply following the dietary and supplement recommendations. Or you may need to include herbal extracts. Whatever it takes to ease your PMS and steady the hormonal tumult, remember this: You are embarking on a lifestyle change that can make you feel and look great!

Understand PMS first

A diagnosis of PMS is based on the existence of four conditions:

· A woman's symptoms must correspond with the luteal phase of the menstrual cycle (that is the last 14 days of her cycle, or 14 days before her period starts);

· Symptoms must be absent during the follicular phase of the menstrual cycle (the first 14 days of her cycle, including when she is bleeding);

· Symptoms recur almost every month, and must be severe enough to interfere with some aspect of her lifestyle.

· The timing of the appearance and disappearance of symptoms, rather than the presence of specific symptoms, is most important in diagnosing PMS.

Although there are many theories as to why woman experience PMS, hormonal imbalance is the most common culprit. An imbalance may occur because of estrogen overproduction, or because of a relative increase in estrogen due to low progesterone secretion, or other reasons.

Did you know that nutritional deficiencies and liver dysfunction also lead to PMS? A shortage of magnesium and B vitamins can sabotage the liver's ability to clear excess estrogen out of the body. Remember, there is a strong diet/PMS connection. Toxins in the diet, such as alcohol, sugar, caffeine, fatty foods, as well as external sources of estrogen (meat and dairy products, environmental pollutants, as well as foods commercially grown using synthetic pesticides and fertilizers), can compromise liver function and intensify symptoms.

> Conventional treatments for PMS generally address the symptoms only.

Pharmaceuticals for PMS – The trouble with conventional treatments

Conventional treatments for PMS generally address the symptoms only. For example, a woman who experiences irritability, nervousness, and lack of control may be prescribed a tranquilizer. A woman who suffers from premenstrual depression may be given Prozac®, a popular antidepressant.

Two examples of common, conventional approaches to PMS, and their potential dangers.

1. Antidepressants (Prozac®): Antidepressant drugs are becoming the primary conventional treatment for PMS. Drugs like Prozac are used to treat major forms of depression. It increases the levels of certain brain chemicals that may improve mood. It does not treat the underlying cause of PMS-hormone and nutritional imbalances. Side effects of Prozac can include decreased appetite, weight loss, allergic reactions, headaches, nervousness, insomnia, drowsiness, tremors, dizziness, fatigue, impaired concentration, altered taste, nausea, vomiting, diarrhea, hair loss, and suicidal thoughts.

> Nature has provided herbs and foods for natural hormone balancing and herbal medicines are among the safest and most effective therapies for PMS.

2. Birth Control Pills: These drugs are primarily used to suppress ovulation. However they have powerful side effects including, but not limited to: fluid retention, weight gain, breakthrough bleeding (spotting in the middle of menstrual cycle), altered menstrual pattern, lack of menstruation (during and following cessation of drug), increased susceptibility to yeast infection of the genital tissues, hypertension, intensification of migraine-like headaches, and intensification of fibrocystic breast changes.

Studies indicate that women over 30 years of age who smoke and use oral contraceptives increase their risk of heart attack significantly. A woman should not take these drugs if she has a history of thrombophlebitis, embolism, heart attack, stroke, breast cancer, impaired liver function, abnormal and unexplained vaginal bleeding, or sickle cell disease. Additionally, birth control pills are contraindicated in liver disease, and long-term use requires a physician's supervision and evaluation every six months.

Nature's top herbal solutions: a better way

There is a better way. Nature has provided herbs and foods for natural hormone balancing and herbal medicines are among the safest and most effective therapies for PMS.

Balance those hormones with Vitex

Vitex (Agnus-castus) is the most popular herbal remedy for PMS. Although vitex as a supplement does not supply hormones, it does act directly on the hypo-thalamus and pituitary gland. These organs control the secretion of the follicle-stimulating hormones (FSH) and luteinizing hormones (LH) that control production of estrogen and progesterone. Vitex stimulates the hypothalamus and pituitary to increase LH levels and slightly decrease FSH levels. This action leads to an increase of progesterone and a balancing effect between estrogen and progesterone.

Vitex also reduces high levels of the hormone prolactin. High levels of this hormone can cause breast tenderness. Reducing abnormally high prolactin can improve symptoms of PMS.

The science behind Vitex

Many clinical trials have demonstrated vitex's ability to relieve PMS. Its clinical value has been well documented in a monograph by the prestigious German Commission E (medical council that analyzes herbal medicines in Germany). Studies have demonstrated that vitex supplementation can reduce physical complaints (such as headaches, breast tenderness, bloating, fatigue, and sweet cravings), and psychological complaints (such as anxiety, irritability, depression, mood swings, and a lack of concentration) after using vitex extract for a minimum of one month. In two surveys, gynecology clinics in Germany looked at 1,500 women for an average of 166 days. The women took 40 drops of vitex extract tincture every morning. Both the physicians and patients used questionnaires to rate the treatment. Fifty-seven percent of the patients reported improvement, and 33 percent reported complete relief of PMS symptoms. The physicians' ratings were positive 92 percent of the time.

An additional study has demonstrated that vitex reduced prolactin levels and normalized progesterone levels in women with high levels of the hormone prolactin in the blood.

Side effects: Rare. Mild digestive upset and skin rash have been reported in fewer than two percent of the women monitored while taking vitex. This botanical is safe to use, except during pregnancy.

Note: Vitex is usually taken for three to five months to correct underlying hormonal imbalances and to resolve PMS. Average dosage is 40 drops of tincture, or 160 to 240 mg of standardized capsule extract daily.

Bloated and puffy? Take care of water retention

Potassium-rich dandelion leaves (Taraxacum officinale) are one of the best natural diuretics available. This herb is useful for the water retention and uncomfortable bloating so typical of PMS. Dandelion's diuretic activity compares well to Lasix®, a popular pharmacological diuretic. Unlike Lasix®, dandelion does not deplete potassium. As a safe and effective diuretic, dandelion helps the kidneys to gently eliminate excess water and toxins. Dandelion leaves also provide additional nutritional support as they are an excellent source of vitamin A and are richer in calcium, iron, magnesium and fiber than either broccoli or spinach. Dandelion effectively reduces the uncomfortable bloating and swelling that many women experience during the last seven to 14 days of their menstrual cycle.

Side effects: None have been reported.

PMS making you anxious and irritable?

Passionflower (Passiflora incarnata) a calming and relaxing botanical nervine, gently address the restlessness, irritability and insomnia that so often accompanies PMS. Its key actions are sedative and antispasmodic. As a mild, nonaddictive herbal nerve relaxer, it is calming and reduces anxiety, and is frequently used for insomnia. It does not make a person sleepy; rather, it works by reducing the tension and anxiety that prevent sleep. It is safe and free of side effects. In our clinical practice we have had much success using passionflower.

Experts feel that various flavonoids in passionflower are responsible for its relaxing and anti-anxiety benefits. Clinically, passionflower is a valuable adjunct in the treatment of the emotional instability associated with PMS. According to herbalist Daniel Mowrey. "Passionflower is frequently used in the treatment of dysmenorrhea (painful menstruation), PMS, pelvic atony (lack of tone), and for allaying the general nervousness that sometimes accompanies the menstrual cycle."

Side effects: None

What can we do about painful cramps and breast tenderness?

Dong quai (Angelica sinensis also known as Tang-Kuei, Dang Gui) has been used in traditional Chinese medicine to treat gynecological ailments, such as irregular menses, painful menses, amenorrhea (no menses), and related pain. Dong quai reduces breast tenderness and relieves cramps by relaxing the smooth muscles of the uterus. In animal studies, Dong quai protects and increases liver metabolism. Although there is confusion in the literature as to whether Dong quai has a phytoestrogen effect, it nonetheless has a rich history of hormone balancing.

Side effects: Low toxicity. Fair-skinned individuals may become more sensitive to light and sunshine. For a small number of women this herb may increase bleeding if taken during the menstrual flow. So I suggest not using the herb while on your period.

The PMS herbal formula—it really works!

My husband and I designed the following formula and tested it in our clinic. We recommend this formula to our patients with PMS. Because their symptoms disappear, many women find that after taking the formula for three to five months, they no longer need to use it, or may use it only occasionally.

Dosage per capsule:

Vitex (Chasteberry) (0.6% Aucubine) 120mg

Dandelion leaf 4:1 extract (3% Vitexine) ..80mg

Passionflower 4:1 extract 80mg

Dong quai 8:1 extract (0.8% Ligustilide) ...50mg

Directions: Take 2 capsules daily, except during your period. If you are pregnant or breast-feeding, consult a physician trained in natural medicine before using any herbs.

Herbs for a healthy liver

A healthy liver is important to efficiently metabolize hormones. By optimizing liver function, a woman can reduce and prevent PMS symptoms. Beneficial herbs for the liver include dandelion root, milk thistle, burdock root, chicory, and bupleurum. We recommend supplementing one or more of these herbs for six weeks to optimize liver health.

Superior dandelion root

We have already discussed dandelion leaf, but dandelion root is also a great herb to improve liver health and treat PMS. Dandelion root is so helpful it deserves extra attention. Dandelion root stimulates the flow of bile in the liver and gallbladder. Bile is one of the major routes used to excrete hormone metabolites and toxins. They go into the stool and out of the body. Optimizing bile flow improves liver health, and ultimately, hormone balance. According to noted herbalist Rosemary Gladstar, "The root is considered the herb par excellence for the liver and is used for all liver disorders, digestive upsets, and gallbladder problems." Dandelion also benefits the female reproductive system, by helping to regulate and normalize hormone production.

Eat fresh, organic plant-based foods

Proper diet and nutrition are essential for correcting the under-lying hormonal imbalances and nutritional deficiencies of PMS. Vegetables, fruits, whole grains, legumes, herbs, nuts, and seeds are the main components of a plant-based diet. Eat fresh, organic foods. Try to avoid processed foods. It has been shown that vegetarian women have much less circulating free estrogen in their blood than non-vegetarian women. A diet focused on plant foods, vegetarian or not, leads to less circulating estrogen, decreasing one's susceptibility to PMS and can also reduce your risk of many serious, potentially life-threatening diseases, such as cancer and cardiovascular disease.

Proper diet and nutrition are essential for correcting the underlying hormonal imbalances and nutritional deficiencies of PMS.

Think high fiber

Vegetarians' higher fiber intake is believed to be one of the main reasons for more balanced estrogen levels. Fiber helps expel fecal waste from the colon. It also helps clear out the hormone estrogen. Many studies suggest that high-fiber diets help reduce PMS symptoms.

Soy—Food as medicine

Most nutritionally oriented physicians advise women of all ages to increase their consumption of soy. The phytoestrogens in soy have a balancing effect on estrogen receptors at the cell surface. If estrogen levels are too high, then soy isoflavones block estrogen uptake at the cellular level. This hormone-balancing effect helps ward off PMS symptoms. Soy isoflavone extracts are also available as supplements.

Liver-healthy foods?

Proper hormone metabolism depends on a healthy liver. Consume foods that support the liver such as carrots, dandelion greens, burdock root, beets, mustard greens, black radish, apples and saffron, watercress, beets, parsley, artichokes, cherries, grapefruit, parsnips, endive garlic, and onion. Fresh fruit and vegetable juicing is also a good idea. The high vitamin, mineral, phytochemical, and chlorophyll content of these foods are very beneficial for the liver. In addition, drink at least six 8-ounce glasses of purified water daily to flush toxins from the liver and the rest of the body.

Reduce saturated fats and sweets

A diet low in saturated fat, found in red meat and dairy products, helps reduce estrogen levels. Also, non-organic meat contains traces of estrogen and other hormones from livestock that have been injected with these substances. Avoid harmful fats, such as trans-fatty acids found in margarine and partially hydrogenated oils. Women following a low-fat diet have been shown to experience a reduction in PMS symptoms.

Studies have also shown that women who consume more sugar suffer from more severe PMS symptoms. A study of 853 female university students investigated the impact of a high-sugar diet. Researchers found a strong correlation between high sugar consumption and PMS.

Pass on the salt shaker, the caffeine and alcohol

If water retention is a problem, restrict your use of salt. Increase your intake of potassium, found in fresh fruits and vegetables. High salt intake combined with low potassium can lead to water retention and high blood pressure.

Caffeine worsens PMS symptoms such as anxiety, depression, and breast tenderness. Long-term use of caffeine, in coffee, soft drinks, chocolate, and some pain relievers for example, leads to fatigue, adrenal exhaustion, and thus depression. Also, too much caffeine is toxic to the liver. Even more than sugar, alcohol depletes B vitamins, magnesium, zinc, and damages liver cells. This interferes with the proper metabolism of hormones. We know it's hard but try turning to herbal teas, such as peppermint and chamomile, for a refreshing beverage.

Vitamins and minerals to the rescue

Specific nutritional supplements have proven valuable in controlling PMS symptoms. Interestingly, most of them work by improving the liver's ability to clear estrogen out of the body.

The Vitamin B6 connection

Caffeine worsens PMS symptoms such as anxiety, depression, and breast tenderness.

Vitamin B6 is one of the most important supplements in the treatment and prevention of PMS. It is a cofactor in the breakdown of estrogen in the liver and in the synthesis of neurotransmitters, such as serotonin and norepinephrine (brain chemicals that elevate mood). It also helps regulate hormone pathways.

Vitamin B6 works synergistically with magnesium. In one double-blind, crossover trial, 84 percent of the women undergoing vitamin B6 treatment experienced a reduction of PMS symptoms, specifically headaches, swelling, bloating, depression, and irritability.

Recommended dosage: 50 to 100 mg in divided doses, or a B-complex formula. Many multivitamins contain sufficient vitamin B6.

Calcium

A study that determined the effectiveness of calcium on PMS was published in the American Journal of Obstetrics and Gynecologists in August of 1998. Women received 1200 mg of calcium carbonate daily or a placebo for three menstrual cycles. There was a significant reduction in PMS symptoms by the second and third menstrual cycle in women taking the calcium versus women taking the placebo. Researchers concluded "calcium supplementation is a simple and effective treatment in premenstrual syndrome, resulting in a major reduction in overall luteal phase symptoms."

Could it be a magnesium deficiency?

A magnesium deficiency can account for many PMS symptoms. Studies have shown that PMS sufferers have lower levels of magnesium in their red blood cells, compared to women without PMS.

Magnesium works as a cofactor in the synthesis of dopamine, an important neurotransmitter (related to the nervous system); as a cofactor involved in the breakdown of estrogen; in the synthesis of prostaglandins (which regulate hormone pathways by activating vitamin B6 in energy production. The use of diuretics (and other prescription drugs), alcohol, high fat intake, dairy products, stress, and malabsorption can all deplete the body's stores of magnesium.

Recommended dosage: 250 to 500 mg daily. This may be included in a general multivitamin, a woman's multivitamin, or a calcium/magnesium supplement.

Zinc—a natural way to lower prolactin

High prolactin levels are associated with PMS. Zinc helps balance and lower these abnormally high prolactin levels.

Recommended dosage: 15 to 30 mg daily. This may be included in a general multivitamin or a woman's multivitamin.

Help tender, painful breasts with Evening Primrose Oil & Vitamin E

Evening primrose oil is a dietary source of GLA, an essential fatty acid. GLA is a precursor to prostaglandins, which have a regulating effect on hormones and other body systems. Studies show that evening primrose oil supplementation may help PMS-related depression, irritability, breast pain and tenderness, and fluid retention.

Since essential fatty acids are important to hormonal health, I recommend that all my patients take omega 3 fatty acids (flaxseeds and flaxseed oil, fish and fish oils) along with their omega 6 (eg. evening primrose) supplements.

Recommended dosage: 2,000 to 3,000 mg of Evening Primrose Oil that contains approximately 200 to 300 mg of GLA.

Another good option is an oil blend that includes omega-3 fatty and omega-6 fatty acids (GLA).

Vitamin E helps effectively reduce breast tenderness associated with PMS. It has also been shown to significantly reduce other PMS symptoms.

Recommended dosage: 400 to 800 IU daily. Natural vitamin E (d-alpha-tocopherol), with a blend of mixed tocopherols, is best.

Natural progesterone—when other therapies are not enough

Natural progesterone is an option for the treatment of PMS. We recommend its use when dietary, herbal, and supplement therapies are not enough. It is normally used after ovulation until the period starts.

Could it be the thyroid?

Studies show that many women with PMS have low thyroid activity. When these women took thyroid hormone, their PMS symptoms were resolved. Have a physician check your thyroid function. If your thyroid gland is under-functioning, we recommend using natural thyroid. Interestingly, thyroid function may return to normal when hormone balance is achieved.

Incorporate exercise

As with many health conditions, exercise reduces and prevents PMS symptoms, especially depression.

See your physician before starting any exercise program. The most important factor in starting and sticking with an exercise routine is finding an activity you enjoy.

Try the natural way first

Without question, natural therapies for PMS should be tried before considering pharmaceutical medications. Underlying hormonal imbalances usually respond well to herbal, nutritional, and other natural therapies. A three-month treatment period is recommended when following natural protocols. Consult a holistic healthcare practitioner for further guidance and an individualized treatment plan or contact us at the Natural Physician Team of Dr. Angela and Dr. Mark Stengler at *www.thenaturalphysician.com* or *www.naturalfactors.com*

CHAPTER 2

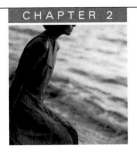

Are You Approaching Menopause?

For some women the transition to menopause can begin as early as age thirty-five. Periods become heavier or lighter, they can last longer or become a few days shorter. Women who would normally sail through their monthly cycles now get PMS, hot flushes or night sweats. As women get closer to menopause, symptoms become more pronounced. How can women minimize the discomfort as they pass through this milestone? Again, balancing the hormones is the key.

31

"I remember Gloria, a patient I was working with my last year of medical school. She was in menopause and had some very severe symptoms, which included fatigue, depression, circulation problems (her feet would turn bright red and were painfully swollen), hot flashes, poor memory, and various digestive problems. We had been treating her for some time with limited results. While reviewing her case, it dawned on me that the cause of many of her problems was probably hormonal imbalance. Gloria was on conventional hormone (synthetic estrogen and progesterone) replacement from her family doctor. Immediately I looked up the side effects of these synthetic hormones to discover that almost all of her symptoms were listed as side effects! This correlated with many of her health problems, which happened to begin around the time she began these hormones. I suggested to my medical school supervisor that we should get her off the synthetic hormones and onto a "natural" herbal hormone balancing therapy. Hesitantly, the supervisor agreed. Gloria returned to the clinic a month later, to everyone's amazement she had tremendous improvement in most of her symptoms. This taught me two valuable points. First, synthetic hormones had the potential to cause serious side effects. Second, natural treatments, such as herbal medicines are very effective and safe in relieving menopausal symptoms. Now, many years later, I always consider hormonal imbalances as a possible contributor to illness in women. I also use natural therapies as the first line of treatment for menopause." Dr. Angela Stengler, ND

First understand what happens to your body

At around 50 years of age, a woman's menstrual cycle usually becomes irregular. Ovulation fails to occur in many of these cycles. Some months or years later the cycle stops altogether and the female sex hormones diminish rapidly. After six to twelve months of no menstrual cycle, a woman has entered menopause.

The menstrual cycle—a dance of hormones

To understand this hormonal change, we must first understand what happens, hormonally, during the 28-day cycle of a regular menstrual cycle.

Days 1-5: Day one of the woman's menstrual cycle is when bleeding begins. The shedding of the endometrial lining of the uterus is caused by a fall in estrogen and progesterone. The decline of these two hormones signals the uterus that pregnancy has not occurred. During this time, FSH (follicle stimulating hormone, a hormone released by the pituitary gland in the brain) rises. FSH is suppressed by estrogen therefore, when estrogen decreases, FSH rises. FSH causes growth of follicles in the ovaries prior to ovulation. By days 5-7, one of the follicles responds to FSH more than the others and starts secreting large amounts of estrogen.

Days 6-14: As estrogen begins to rise, FSH begins to fall. This rise in estrogen stimulates the endometrial lining of the uterus to thicken, in preparation for possible implantation of the fertilized egg.

Day 14: Estrogen helps stimulate a large and sudden release of LH (lutenizing hormone, a hormone released by the pituitary gland to cause ovulation). This LH surge causes the follicle to rupture and the egg is expelled into the fallopian tube.

Days 14-28: During this time, estrogen and progesterone rise and then begin to fall. After the follicle ruptures, and its walls collapse, it is known as a corpus luteum. The corpus luteum begins secreting large amounts of progesterone. Progesterone further helps prepare the endometrial lining of the uterus for implantation of the fertilized egg. If the egg is not fertilized, the corpus luteum continues to release hormone until it runs out. Without these hormones, the uterus sheds its lining. Since estrogen has fallen, FSH levels start to rise and the hormonal dance begins again.

Before and after menopause

In the lifetime of a menstruating woman, estrogen, progesterone, FSH and LH are in a delicate balance. During the years before menopause (perimenopause), estrogen and/or progesterone cycle at lower levels, causing FSH and/or LH to be released at a higher level (in an attempt to increase estrogen and/or progesterone). This is the time a woman experiences irregular cycles. After menopause there is a continuously high level of FSH and consistently low levels of estrogen and progesterone. This occurs because the follicles remaining in the ovaries of a perimenopausal woman are less sensitive to stimulation by FSH. When a follicle does not develop properly, it secretes less estrogen, failing to suppress the secretion of FSH by the pituitary gland. Therefore, FSH levels continue to rise. In addition, this low level of estrogen may fail to trigger the LH surge that is responsible for the release of the follicle (ovulation). Since the follicle has not ruptured, it cannot release progesterone. This lowered level of estrogen and progesterone can lead to shortened menstrual cycles. The uterus is being signaled to shed its lining early. Shorter cycles as well as irregular cycles are usually the first signs that perimenopause has started. At the time of menopause, a woman must adjust to the lower levels of estrogen and progesterone in her body.

Have you had these symptoms?

Each woman has a different experience during menopause. The following list contains the most common signs and symptoms associated with this period of hormonal change.

Hot flashes
Mood swings
Depression
Sleep disturbance
Nightsweats
Irregular menses

Decreased libido
Vaginal dryness
Urinary tract infections
Forgetfulness
Heart palpitations
Hypoglycemia
Nausea
Dry skin
Hair loss
High blood pressure
High cholesterol and lipids

Menopause-two health conditions to be aware of

Osteoporosis and heart disease are two conditions that become an increased threat to women as they enter menopause. In osteoporosis, the bones become thin and weak, leading to a susceptibility to fractures. Though the beginnings of osteoporosis can begin as a child, bone loss accelerates after menopause possibly due to the decrease in estrogen and progesterone. In addition, the risk of heart disease substantially increases as a woman enters menopause. These two conditions make it even more important to follow the diet, supplement and herbal guidelines that are outlined below.

The potential dangers of synthetic hormones

The risks associated with pharmaceutical treatment and the scientific validation of many natural therapies are leading reasons as to why women are turning toward natural medicine. As a matter of fact, close to fifty percent of women who use pharmaceutical hormones for menopause discontinue its use on their own due to side effects or the fear of side effects.

The many functions of a horse

Did you know that horses are not just for horseback riding? Believe it or not, the most commonly prescribed form of synthetic estrogen comes from pregnant mare's urine! Hence the term 'Premarin®.' In a woman's body, estrogen is found in three forms: estriol 60-80%, estrone 10-20%, and estradiol 10-20%. Horses' urine (Premarin®), is composed of estrone 75-80%, equilin 6-15% (a form of estrogen not found in humans), and estradiol and others 5-19%. As you can see, there is incompatibility between natural estrogens found in the woman's body and Premarin®. When physicians trained in natural medicine prescribe natural estrogens for the treatment of menopausal symptoms, they use the ratios and forms of estrogens found in the female body. Better still, herbal medicines are generally the

> Believe it or not, the most commonly prescribed form of synthetic estrogen comes from pregnant mare's urine! Hence the term 'Premarin®.'

best choice in treating menopause due to their compatibility with the body's hormone receptors.

Premarin® and the estrogen patch are forms of synthetic estrogen with potentially dangerous side effects.

Just read the PDR, (Physicians' Desk Reference). Synthetic estrogen side effects include but are not limited to: withdrawal bleeding, fluid retention, bloating, headache, nausea, vomiting, gallbladder disease, blood clots, anxiety/irritability, vaginal discharge, breast tenderness/enlargement, spotty darkening of the skin, enlarged uterine fibroids, endometrial cancer, and breast cancer.

Provera®, synthetic progestin, has its own side effects. According to Dr. John Lee, a retired medical doctor who specialized in gynecology and an expert on hormone therapy, the potential side effects of Provera include fluid retention, epilepsy, migraine headaches, asthma, heart or kidney dysfunction, breakthrough menstrual bleeding and irregularities, depression, decreased glucose tolerance, blood clots, breast tenderness, galactorrea, allergic skin rashes, acne, hair loss or hair growth, swelling/edema, weight changes, changes in cervical secretions, jaundice, insomnia, thrombophlebitis, and pulmonary embolism.

Unfortunately, it appears that synthetic hormones were designed for profit, not healing.

Unfortunately, it appears that synthetic hormones were designed for profit, not healing. For pharmaceutical companies to patent a hormone, and thus control its sale, it must not be identical to what is naturally found in the body. Therefore, for a patent to be approved, a chemical alteration must have taken place. As may be expected, problems arise because the cell receptors in the body are designed to interact with the hormones naturally produced by the body. Similar to a lock and key, with the hormone being the key and the lock being the cell receptor, a mismatched key (in this case the synthetic hormone), will not fit properly into the lock. Plant substances such as phytoestrogens, are bio-identical to the body's hormones and act to potentiate instead of replacing the body's hormones.

Are you at high risk? Know your treatment options

What type of approach should you use to alleviate your menopausal symptoms? Ultimately, it's your decision. Here are some guidelines to help you. Discuss any treatment program with your physician. A naturopathic physician is an excellent resource.

Low Risk:

Normal physiologic menopause (not induced by medications, surgery or other health conditions) around the age of 45-55 years

No family history of cardiovascular disease or osteoporosis

No long-term use of medications that lead to increased risk of cardiovascular disease or osteoporosis

Medium to heavy frame

Non-smoker, healthy diet, weight bearing and aerobic exercises at least 3 times a week, alcohol consumption less than three times weekly.

Treatment recommendations:

If you have no menopausal symptoms: See sections on diet, exercise, and supplements.

For mild to moderate symptoms of menopause try herbal medicine, diet, exercise, and supplements.

For severe symptoms consider natural progesterone and/or natural hormone replacement.

Medium Risk:

Normal physiologic menopause around the age of 45 to 55 years and any one or two of the following:

Family history of cardiovascular disease or osteoporosis

Small, slender, Caucasian

Smoker; significant smoking history

History of oligomenorrhea (too few menses) or amenorrhea (no menstrual cycle)

History of stress fractures

Long term use of medication associated with osteoporosis risk (e.g. Prednisone)

Systemic diseases associated with osteoporosis

Mild hyperlipidemia (high blood cholesterol and fats) plus high blood pressure

75-80% bone density

Moderate alcohol intake (three times a week)

Sedentary life plus poor diet

Treatment recommendations:

No menopausal symptoms: See sections on diet, exercise, and supplements. Consider use of natural progesterone.

For mild to moderate symptoms of menopause try herbal medicine, diet, and supplements. Consider use of natural progesterone and/or natural hormone replacement.

High Risk:

If your doctor has diagnosed you with a high risk for osteoporosis or heart disease, consider using natural progesterone, with natural estrogen replacement.

Many new studies are revealing that synthetic estrogen plus progestin (synthetic progesterone) is not effective for postmenopausal women who have heart disease. One such study, known as the HERS study , published in JAMA in August of 1998, found that after four years of treatment with synthetic estrogen and progestin, the overall rate of coronary heart disease events (including heart attacks) in postmenopausal women with established coronary disease was not reduced. This treatment did , however, increase the rate of blood clots and gallbladder disease. Researchers state "Based on the finding of no overall cardiovascular benefit and a pattern of early increase in risk of coronary heart disease events, we do not recommend starting this treatment for the purpose of secondary prevention of coronary heart disease."

Nature's top herbs for menopause

Herbal medicines are one of the safest and most effective therapies to ease the transition through menopause. Their use has been documented through thousands of years.

One of the unique aspects of hormone balancing herbs is their phytoestrogens or plant estrogens component. Rather than exerting a drug-like action, phytoestrogens tonify and balance the glandular system of women (and males too). Side effects are not an issue as these phytoestrogens work in harmony with your body's hormones. Phytoestrogens may exert weak estrogenic effects (up to 2% as strong as estrogen). They have a balancing or amphoteric action in the body.

The balancing effect of phytoestrogens

This amphoteric effect refers to the ability of phytoestrogens to bind to and block estrogen receptors if estrogen levels are too high, or enhance cellular uptake of estrogen if levels are too low. Due to this balancing effect, many phytoestrogenic herbs can be used for conditions that involve estrogen excess such as PMS, or estrogen deficiency such as menopause. Another benefit of phytoestrogens is their role in cancer prevention. Studies in animals have shown the effectiveness of phytoestrogens in inhibiting breast tumors.

Herbal medicines are one of the safest and most effective therapies to ease the transition through menopause. Their use has been documented through thousands of years.

Most herbal formulas that alleviate menopausal symptoms are rich in phytoestrogens. Here are the top herbal medicines for menopause.

Black Cohosh

Many clinical trials have demonstrated the efficacy of black cohosh (Cimicifuga racemosa) for the relief of menopausal symptoms. Black cohosh is the most popular and potent Western herb for the treatment of menopause. Its clinical value has been well documented by the prestigious German Commission E monograph.

Black cohosh inhibits receptor sites in the pituitary gland and hypothalamus. A large open study followed 629 menopausal women who supplemented 80 mg of black cohosh extract for six to eight weeks. Most of the women noticed beneficial results within four weeks of beginning treatment. Within eight weeks, a large percentage of women reported complete resolution of symptoms. The treatment was well tolerated with only 7% of patients reporting mild digestive upset. Refer to Table 1 for these amazing results.

Side effects: There is no known toxicity with black cohosh. Clinical studies on over 1700 patients over a three to six month period showed excellent tolerance. Extremely high doses may cause digestive upset, headaches, and dizziness.

Recommended dosage: 40 mg capsule containing a standardized extract of 2.5% triterpene glycosides taken two to four times daily.

Symptom Improvements with Black Cohosh

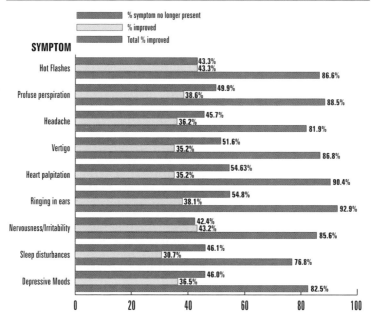

Vitex can help hot flashes

It is believed that menopausal symptoms are improved through an effect on the hypothalamus and pituitary gland by altering FSH and LH secretion. Vitex appears to increase LH secretion, leading to increased progesterone levels. Low progesterone levels contribute significantly to menopausal symptoms. In a recent clinical study, women taking vitex experienced relief of menopausal symptoms. European physicians commonly recommend vitex for the treatment of hot flashes.

Side effects: Rare. Mild digestive upset and skin rash have been reported in less than two percent of the women monitored while supplementing vitex.

Recommended dosage: (6:1 concentration) 80 mg twice daily of a standardized extract of 0.6% aucubin. Tincture dosage is 40 drops one to two times daily.

Balance estrogen with Wild Yam Root

Wild Yam (Dioscorea villosa) does not supply progesterone. However, as a phytoestrogen it may help balance estrogen and progesterone levels in the body. It has also been shown to lower triglycerides (fats) and raise HDL (good) cholesterol. Wild yam contains the steroidal saponin known as diosgenin. Diosgenin acts as the precursor for the pharmaceutical synthesis of estrogen, progesterone, and pregnenolone.

Note: The body does not convert diosgenin into hormones such as pregnenolone and progesterone. This is done only through chemical synthesis in a laboratory. Wild yam roots also has anti-spasmodic, anti-inflammatory, and nerve relaxant properties.

Side effects: Non-toxic, although large amounts may cause nausea.

Recommended dosage: (10:1 concentration) 75 mg twice daily.

Licorice Root—a gift from Traditional Chinese Medicine

One of the most important herbs in traditional Chinese medicine, licorice (Glycyrrhiza uralensis) has also been used in Western herbal therapy (Glycyrrhiza glabra) to treat menopause, PMS, respiratory infections, and digestive inflammatory conditions such as ulcers. Licorice has a balancing action on estrogen and progesterone and supports adrenal gland function. These glands produce estrogen and progesterone after the ovaries fail to respond to FSH and LH.

Side effects: Sensitive persons may experience water retention and an increase in blood pressure at high dosages.

Recommended dosage: 4:1 concentration of 75 mg twice daily.

Two-fold help with Hops

Hops (Humulus lupulus) are powerful phytoestrogens. According to herbalist Rosemary Gladstar, "Hops contain high concentrations of plant hormones that have estrogen-like effects on the female system." This phytoestrogen effect balances estrogen levels in the body. As a nerve tonic hops help calm the nerves and treat imbalances due to stress and nervousness.

Side effects: No known side effects taking hops internally.

Recommended dosage: 5:1 concentration at 25 mg twice daily.

The menopause formula—combining the best

Single herbs such as black cohosh can be used alone to treat menopause. However, best results are achieved by combining a variety of herbs. Each herb has a different action on the body so a synergistic combination can treat more symptoms. One of the oldest (more than 2,000 years) and most developed systems is Oriental Medicine, where single herbs are rarely used to treat a condition. A blend of indicated herbs is always preferred.

As a naturopathic physician, I have had a lot of success helping women ease the symptoms of this life change. Based on current scientific research and clinical experience, I developed an herbal formula that helps women from the beginning of perimenopause through menopause while they avoid the risks that come with hormone replacement therapy. Each herb chosen exerts a balancing effect on hormones, and reduces unpleasant symptoms. Consider the herbs in the Natural Factors® Menopause Formula.

Dosage per capsule:

Vitex Extract 12:1 ....80mg
Wild Yam Extract 10:1 ....75mg
Licorice Root Extract 4:1 ....75mg
Black Cohosh Extract 6:1........................40mg
Hops Extract 5:1......................................25mg

Directions: Take 1 capsule twice daily before meals.

If symptoms persist after one month increase the dosage to three or four capsules daily.

Choosing the right supplements

You can achieve tremendous health benefits from dietary supplements.

High Potency Multivitamin without iron –provides a complete profile of vitamins and minerals to prevent illness. If you have iron-deficiency anemia, ask your physician about iron supplements.

Calcium/Magnesium Citrate–can help prevent and treat osteoporosis. A total of 1,000 mg a day is recommended for strong bones. Look for formulas that contain a blend of bone-building nutrients.

Natural Vitamin E (d-alpha-tocopherol) 400 to 800 IU daily of mixed tocopherols for cardiovascular protection.

Essential Fatty Acids are found flaxseeds and flaxseed oil, evening primrose oil, fish oil, or a blend of essential fatty acids. It is best to use a blend like Natural Factors Omega Factors.

Ease the transition with diet

Proper diet and nutrition are essential as you make the transition through menopause. The foods we list in this section will not only help in reducing your menopausal symptoms; they may reduce your risk of conditions such as cancer and cardiovascular disease.

Eat a plant based diet

Vegetables, fruits, grains, legumes, herbs, nuts, and seeds are the main components of a plant-based diet. Eat fresh, organic foods. Try to eat primarily unprocessed foods such as whole grains.

Eat your vegetables but here's an option

If you are not eating fruits and vegetables regularly, consider a daily Greens Drink to enrich your diet. They are composed of super green foods such as barley grass, wheat grass, alfalfa, and others. They also contain enzymes, disease fighting phytochemicals, and chlorophyll (a potent detoxifier) that are not found in vitamin formulas. For more information on the health benefits of super green foods see the book *Drink Your Greens* (Impakt Publications 1998).

Try to minimize these foods:

· Red meat and poultry due to hormone content (unless organic).

· Dairy products due to hormone content (unless organic).

· Refined sugar products can weaken the immune system and promote cardiovascular disease.

· Fried foods are hard to digest and they can damage the cardiovascular and immune systems. Steam, bake, broil, or poach when possible.

· Preservatives, artificial colorings, and other food additives damage the immune system.

If you are not eating fruits and vegetables regularly, consider a daily Greens Drink to enrich your diet.

· Caffeine depletes calcium and other minerals, irritates the digestive tract, and can overwhelm the adrenal (i.e. stress) glands.

· Salt may throw potassium levels out of balance and can trigger high blood pressure. Soft drinks contain phosphoric acid which depletes calcium.

· Alcohol depletes calcium and other minerals and increases cancer risk. Small amounts of red wine are fine, although unsweetened, organic grape juice provides the same benefits for the cardiovascular system.

We can't say enough about exercise

Regular exercise is important to a healthy lifestyle before, during and after menopause. Regular exercise reduces hot flashes, increases bone density, strength and resiliency, and reduces the risk of cardiovascular disease. Exercises such as walking, jogging, aerobics, tennis, swimming, cycling are important for heart and bone health. Find an activity that you enjoy. Exercise for 30 minutes at least three times a week for optimal benefits. If you've been inactive, see your physician before starting any exercise routine.

Benefit from natural, not synthetic, hormones

Herbal therapy, diet, exercise, and supplements are the first line of treatment for menopausal symptoms. Some women may need hormone replacement therapy—due to severe menopausal symptoms or a high risk factor for osteoporosis. We do not advocate synthetic hormones of any type, such as Premarin® or Provera®. Instead, talk with your holistic physician about the use of natural estrogen and natural progesterone. Every case is different. Some women may also need hormones such as DHEA, testosterone, and thyroid.

Menopause is not a disease

Menopause is a natural transition for women. In many cultures women look forward to menopause, primarily as a relief from childbearing. In these cultures the symptoms of menopause are much less frequent. Most symptoms can be alleviated with natural methods such as herbs, nutrition, supplements, and exercise. If you do need hormone replacement therapy consult a holistic health practitioner to help you determine what is best for you.

More to learn

We recommend three outstanding books on this topic:

Natural Woman, Natural Menopause by Marcus Laux ND and Christine Conrad (Harper Collins)

Natural Hormone Replacement by Jonathan Wright MD and John Morgenthaler (Smart Publications)

What Your Doctor May Not Tell You About Menopause by John R. Lee MD (Warner Books)

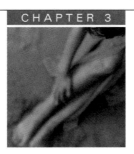

CHAPTER 3

Healthy Bones for a Lifetime

You've reached menopause. Now's the time to talk to your doctor about osteoporosis. However, it is necessary to maximize bone health and prevent bone loss long before menopause.

Too many women come to our office with osteoporosis. This debilitating condition restricts their lives. Although most women know that they need to increase their calcium intake, few know what they can do to prevent and possibly reverse osteoporosis. Menopause does not mean you'll automatically develop osteoporosis. However, it does mean you must research your family, medical, and lifestyle history and decide what you need to do to protect your bones. This information is not only important for adults, but should also be discussed with teenagers.

What is osteoporosis?

Osteoporosis is a reduction in bone mass, causing skeletal weakness and increased susceptibility to bone fractures. In the body, specialized cells, known as osteoclasts, work to resorb (i.e., break down and reabsorb) bone. Other cells, known as osteoblasts, work to form bone. These cells, working together, allow bone to remake itself, to withstand stresses and strains, and to quickly respond to and repair damage.

During growth spurts, more bone is synthesized than is resorbed. However, as we age, more bone is resorbed than is synthesized. The lack of bone formation ultimately results in excessive bone loss.

This condition affects more than 25 million people in North America, and is responsible for over one million bone fractures each year. Bone mass increases from the day we are born, until we reach a maximum density. This is usually age 30 for cortical hone (long bones, such as the arm and leg bones) and age 35 for trabecular bone (found at the ends of long bones, and including the vertebrae, pelvis, and heel). After the mid-30s, bone mass decline until menopause. This abrupt decline suggests that sex hormones play a large role in bone health.

Menopausal women need to know about two types of osteoporosis: Type I osteoporosis (also known as postmenopausal osteoporosis) occurs between the ages of 51 and 75. It is six times more common in women than in men. Type I osteoporosis is largely responsible for bone fractures of the back and wrist. Postmenopausal endocrine (hormone) changes are probably responsible for this condition.

> Since osteoporosis is the most common bone disease in adults, especially in old age, it is important that prevention starts early.

Type II osteoporosis occurs mainly in people over 70 years old. This condition is twice as common in women than men. Type II osteoporosis is a more gradual and age-related condition. Fractures usually occur in the hip, back, arms, below the knee, and pelvis. Age-related reduction in vitamin D synthesis, or resistance to vitamin D activity, may be responsible for this condition. It is important to note that Type I and Type II osteoporosis may occur together in women.

Since osteoporosis is the most common bone disease in adults, especially in old age, it is important that prevention starts early.

Common causes of osteoporosis include lack of physical stress on the bone because of inactivity (not enough weight-bearing exercise), malnutrition, lack of nutrients such as vitamin C (which is necessary for the formation of bone), postmenopausal lack of estrogen secretion (estrogens stimulate bone cells), and old age, a time when growth hormone and other growth factors decrease.

Osteoporosis – it will happen to one in three of us

An estimated one in three women in North America will develop some type of osteoporosis after menopause. Postmenopausal osteoporosis is the cause of 1.3 million fractures each year. To get an idea of how serious this condition is, it is important to note that after a hip fracture, approximately 15 percent of patients die within one year. This is usually because of some complication related to the prolonged immobilization required when a bone is fractured. In addition, 75 percent of patients with hip-fractures lose their independence, and 25 percent require prolonged nursing care. An estimated $7 to $10 billion each year is spent treating complications of osteoporosis. Therefore, if your physician suspects osteoporosis, or if you are monitoring your bone loss, it makes sense to evaluate your bone density.

Risk factors for osteoporosis

Below are the most common, well-documented risk factors associated with osteoporosis. The higher your risk, the more aggressive you need to be for effective prevention and treatment. In addition, the earlier you identify your risk for osteoporosis, the less likely you are to suffer from its consequences. The following list describes the most common risk factors associated with osteoporosis:

- High caffeine intake
- High alcohol intake
- High sugar intake
- Excessive soft drink intake
- High-protein diet (animal protein)
- High salt intake
- Smoking
- Inadequate exercise
- Lack of sun exposure
- Never being pregnant
- Medical conditions
- Postmenopausal
- Premature, surgically induced menopause
- Hyperparathyroidism, hyperthyroidism
- Eating disorders (Anorexia nervosa)
- Type I diabetes
- Rheumatoid arthritis
- Homocysteinemia (excess of homocysteine – a toxic amino acid derivative – in the plasma)
- Liver disease
- Kidney disease
- Cushing's syndrome
- Ankylosing spondylitis
- Connective tissue disease
- Malabsorption
- History of amenorrhea (no menstrual periods; not including when pregnant)
- Surgical resection of the stomach or small intestine
- Genetic
- Caucasian or Asian ethnicity
- Female
- Family member with osteoporosis (mother, grandmother)
- Small body frame
- Medications
- Long-term steroid use (e.g. prednisone)
- Thyroid hormone prescription (too much)
- Lithium
- Chemotherapy
- Heparin (anticoagulant)
- Long-term glucocorticoid therapy
- Long-term use of anti-convulsants

Understanding conventional treatments for osteoporosis

1) Use of synthetic estrogen (for example, conjugated estrogen such as Premarin®, and transdermal estrogen, also known as "the patch") decreases the risk of hip fractures by 50 percent. Early commencement of therapy after menopause and long-term use are recommended. However, the many dangerous side effects of synthetic estrogen are becoming well known to the educated public. In addition, using estrogen without progesterone can lead to serious conditions, such as cancers of the breast and uterus. (See section under "Natural hormone therapy" for safer alternatives.) Also, estrogen only slows down the loss of bone, it does not reverse bone loss.

2) Calcitonin® is a pharmaceutical medication that physicians give patients who cannot take estrogen for the treatment of osteoporosis. Basically, this drug inhibits bone resorption (breakdown and assimilation). Calcitonin® can be given as an injection or a nasal spray. Disadvantages include expense and possible resistance to the drug. Interestingly, actual improvement in fracture rates has not been demonstrated. Furthermore, blood calcium levels must be followed to check for imbalances with this medicine.

3) Fosamax® is another pharmaceutical medication that inhibits bone resorption. This drug is taken orally. Physicians must warn their patients who are taking Fosamax® about the possibility of esophageal irritation. Any pain with swallowing, pain behind the

sternum (upper chest), or pain with speaking must be taken seriously and Fosamax® should be discontinued. Patients must not lie down for 30 minutes after taking Fosamax®, they must swallow it with a full glass of water (six to eight ounces), and they must not take it at bedtime. The risk of severe esophageal irritation is greater if one or more of the aforementioned "rules" are not followed. Patients with active upper gastrointestinal problems (for example, ulcers, inflammation of the stomach or small intestine, difficulty swallowing, or esophageal diseases) should not use Fosamax®, or use it with caution. Daily treatment with Fosamax® is required to maintain the effect of this drug.

4) Evista® is a pharmaceutical medication becoming increasingly popular among menopausal women who have osteoporosis and do not want synthetic hormone therapy. Evista® helps prevent and treat osteoporosis by building and stopping the thinning of bone. It does not increase the risk of uterine or breast cancer. Evista® is not for everyone. If you are pregnant, nursing, have liver problems, or have had blood clots you should not take Evista®. The most serious side effect is blood clots in the veins. The most common side effects are hot flashes and leg cramps from Evista® use.

Bone healthy foods & nutrients

The typical North American diet is detrimental to bone health. Focus on fresh, organic vegetables, fruits, legumes, and whole grains. Combine these foods with fresh fish, lean poultry, and a minimal amount of red meat. Green, leafy vegetables such as collard greens, kale, and lettuce are particularly important. They provide a wealth of vitamins and minerals for bone health, including calcium, vitamin K, boron, and vitamin C. It can be confusing and frustrating to make drastic dietary changes. It's best to keep things simple, take one step at a time, and indulge yourself once in a while. The key is moderation.

> It can be confusing and frustrating to make drastic dietary changes. It's best to keep things simple, take one step at a time, and indulge yourself once in a while.

To improve bone health, one of the major dietary changes you need to make is to reduce animal protein and focus on a plant-based diet. An occasional steak will not harm you. However, a lack of vegetables, grains, legumes, and nuts will.

Some nutritional tips to make it easier

Each week, try to add a food that will support bone health. For example, switch from a low-nutrient salad base, such as iceberg lettuce, to nutrient-rich romaine lettuce. Then, substitute different vegetables each week to your evening salad to achieve a blend of nutrients. Try foods you have never eaten before, such as soy and other beans. Your own innate creativity will help you make appetizing meals. Vegetarian cookbooks are very helpful for plant-based diets.

The problem with coffee, sugar and other cravings

Caffeine promotes the loss of calcium and other bone-building nutrients through the urine. This increases the risk of fractures. In addition to a high sugar and caffeine content, soft drinks are high in phosphoric acid, which leeches calcium from the bone. Try herbal teas and unsweetened fruit juices.

Smoking is a major risk factor for osteoporosis. Do whatever it takes to stop this deadly habit. Natural therapies—such as herbal, homeopathic, and acupuncture treatment programs—can be helpful. The nicotine patch and nicotine gum benefit some people.

Too much protein?

Vegetarian diets are associated with a lower risk of developing osteoporosis. A high-protein diet leads to the urinary excretion of calcium. It is believed that the typical North American high-protein diet is a major factor in the increasing rate of osteoporosis. We recommend protein sources such as fresh fish, legumes, algae sources (such as chlorella, spirulina), and lean poultry.

Why fiber?

Sufficient fiber is essential for your bones and your overall health. Eating more vegetables will add fiber to your diet, necessary for proper elimination. If you don't have regular bowel movements, hormones such as estrogen will continue to be resorbed throughout the body, resulting in imbalances.

Ipriflavone—the cutting edge research

A new natural bone-building substance is making headlines. Called Ipriflavone®, it is isolated from the soy isoflavone daidzein and it holds much promise for the prevention and treatment of osteoporosis. Studies show that it increases bone density and decreases the number of fractures. In an open study, 100 women with osteoporosis were given 200 mg of ipriflavone three times a day for 12 months. The bone density of the 90 women who completed the study increased by 2% after six months and 5.8% after 12 months. I recommend all my patients at risk for osteoporosis take a bone formula containing Ipriflavone® at a dosage of 600 mg daily.

Keep the Calcium & Magnesium coming

Calcium is the most abundant mineral in the body and is constantly flowing in and out of bones. Calcium that the bones lose each day needs to be replaced to prevent demineralization (i.e. loss of bone mass). Osteoporosis involves the loss of calcium and other minerals required for bone structure. Calcium supplementation reduces bone loss in postmenopausal women. The New England Journal of Medicine reported that post-menopausal women who added 1,000 mg of calcium to their normal daily diets experienced a 43 percent reduction in bone loss when compared to controls.

In a study of 169 women, ages 35 to 65, participants were given either a placebo or 1,500 mg of calcium for four years. The group receiving the calcium supplements lost less bone mineral than the placebo group. This study also showed more effect for postmenopausal women versus premenopausal women.

Toxicity: Dosages of 2,000 mg and less are usually well tolerated. Those with hyperparathyroidism (condition caused by an increase in the secretion of the parathyroid – adjacent to the thyroid gland – causing elevated serum calcium) and chronic kidney disease should not supplement calcium without consulting a physician.

Recommended dosage: 1000 - 1200 mg with meals. Calcium citrate, citrate-malate, and hydroxyappatite are all well absorbed. Vitamin D is required for calcium to be absorbed and utilized in the body.

Magnesium—as important as calcium?

Studies show that 39 percent of American women between 15 and 50 years of age have an intake of magnesium that is less than 70 percent of the RDA. Some experts feel this mineral is as important as calcium for bone health. Almost 50 percent of the body's magnesium is found in bones. Magnesium depletion adversely affects bone metabolism, leading to bone fragility. A deficiency of magnesium impairs bone health, since it is needed for proper hormonal activities that control calcium metabolism.

Toxicity: The most common side effect is diarrhea, which goes away when the dosage is reduced. Those with kidney or certain heart conditions should consult a physician before supplementing with magnesium.

Recommended dosage: 500 to 1000 mg of supplemental magnesium daily, with meals.

Want to absorb calcium? You need Vitamin D

Vitamin D promotes calcium absorption through the intestines. It also helps draw calcium from the blood and into the bones. Vitamin D is acquired from foods and when the skin is exposed to the sun. Therefore, those who are indoors all the time risk vitamin D deficiency. This deficiency is common in the elderly.

In one study, 348 women, 70 years and older, received 400 IU of vitamin D or a placebo for two years. Bone density studies revealed an increase of 1.9 percent in the left hip, and 2.6 percent in the right hip for those receiving vitamin D. The placebo group demonstrated decreases of bone density in each hip.

Studies also indicate that the combination of vitamin D and calcium works well. A study of 3,270 female seniors living in nursing homes received 1,200 mg of calcium and 800 IU of vitamin D or placebo. The hip fracture rate was reduced by 43 percent in the group receiving vitamin D and calcium, as compared to placebo.

Toxicity: Persons with hyperparathyroidism or sarcoidosis (a kind of fibrosis) should consult their physician before supplementing. Doses above 1,000 IU may increase blood calcium levels and deposit calcium into the kidneys and internal organs.

Recommended dosage: 400 IU of vitamin D is recommended as a preventative dosage for bone health. For those at risk for osteoporosis, we recommend 400 to 800 IU daily.

Vitamin C for bones and connective tissue

Vitamin C contributes to the formation of collagen, which is involved in bone and connective tissue formation. Studies in animals have shown that a vitamin C deficiency can cause osteoporosis.

Toxicity: Dosages above 2,000 mg can cause diarrhea in some persons. To prevent diarrhea gradually increase the dosage over time.

Recommended dosage: 500 to 1,000 mg daily. Double this dosage if you are a smoker.

Vitamin K activates bone protein

This vitamin activates the bone protein osteocalcin, which holds calcium in the bones. Low vitamin K is associated with osteoporosis and it is important for the healing of fractures.

Toxicity: Those on blood-thinning medications, such as warfarin, should not take supplemental vitamin K.

Recommended dosage: 150 to 500 mcg a day. Supplemental vitamin K cannot be sold in Canada, so we recommend eating green leafy vegetables or use Green Drinks such as Enriching greens as a source of natural vitamin K.

Stronger, harder bones with Manganese

Manganese is needed for healthy bone, skin, and cartilage formation. Manganese stimulates the formation of mucopolysaccharides. These molecules enable calcification (hardening of the bones) to take place.

Toxicity: Dosages and side effects have not yet been established.

Recommended dosage: 4 to 10 mg daily

Silca/silicon

Silica contributes to the formation of collagen. It is also needed as a cofactor in calcification.

Toxicity: Dosages and side effects have not yet been established.

Recommended dosage: 5 to 20 mg of silicon is a safe dosage. Supplemental silicon cannot be sold in Canada, so we recommend a formula with horsetail as a natural source of silica. A dose of 100 to 1,000 mg daily is recommended for silica extract from horsetail (Equisetum arvense).

B vitamins for heart and bones

Vitamin B6, folic acid, and vitamin B12 are all important in the prevention and treatment of osteoporosis. They protect against the buildup of homocysteine, a by-product of protein metabolism. Elevated homocysteine levels may interfere with the formation of collagen, an integral part of bone formation. All three of these B vitamins have been shown to help regulate homocysteine levels. The combination of these three vitamins is more effective than taking any one of them alone.

Recommended dosage: As part of a high-potency multivitamin or B-complex formula:

B6–50 to 100 mg

B12–400 to 1,000 micrograms

Folic acid–400 to 2500 micrograms

Other bone-building agents

The mineral boron plays a special role in bone health. This mineral helps the body utilize vitamin D, reduces urinary excretion of calcium, and increases estrogen production, which slows the loss of bone. There is no RDA, but 1 to 2 mg a day is generally recommended for bone health. It is found in fruits, vegetables, and nuts.

Many vitamins and minerals play a role in bone health. Zinc, copper, strontium, and chromium all are important for bone health. They are usually available in high-quality, high-potency multivitamins. Phosphorous is involved in bone formation, but it is rarely deficient in the diet and seldom needs to be supplemented.

Optimal bone formula

Many of our female patients want to know what supplements to take to help prevent and/or treat osteoporosis. A woman's high-potency multivitamin should include optimal amounts of calcium, magnesium, vitamin D, vitamin C, vitamin K, manganese, silica, B vitamins, and all the other minerals involved with bone health. The combination of the woman's multivitamin and a bone formula should provide a total of 1,000 to 1,200 mg of calcium per day.

An excellent bone formula called Osteo Factors from Natural Factors® contains (per capsule):

Calcium (Citrate) 150mg
Magnesium(Oxide/Citrate) 75mg
Vitamin D3 ....100iu
Ipriflavone...100mg
Vitamin C (Ascorbic Acid) 25mg
Manganese (Citrate) 2mg
Zinc (Citrate) 3mg
Vit. B6 (Pyridoxine HCL) 5mg
Silicon(Horsetail) 0.25mg

Dosage: Take 6 capsules per day. This formula is safe to take on a long term basis.

Importance of digestion

About 40 percent of postmenopausal women have low stomach acid. However, people with low levels of stomach acid absorb significantly less calcium. Adequate levels of stomach acid (hydrochloric acid) are needed for the absorption of minerals such as calcium, magnesium, folic acid, and others. Chronic illness, stress, antacids, nutritional deficiencies, and certain medications can lower stomach acid levels, leading to poor absorption. Supplements such as betaine HCL, and bitter herbs such as gentian root, can be used to increase stomach acid levels. In addition, plant enzymes, taken with meals, can improve intestinal absorption of nutrients.

Note: If you have an ulcer, check with your physician before using any of these digestive supplements.

Let's get moving—building better bones through exercise

Consistent weight-bearing exercise increases bone density. Good forms of weight-bearing exercise include walking, jogging, weightlifting, and racquet sports. Non-weight-bearing exercises, such as swimming, also increase bone density. Any type of exercise that improves coordination and flexibility can reduce the risk of a fall and thus a fracture. One study focused on 200 people, 70 years and older, who followed a regimen of tai chi and computerized balance training for 15 weeks. They had a 47.5 percent reduction in the risk of multiple falls. We recommend 30 minutes of exercise, a minimum of three times a week. Choose activities you enjoy, so you can stick with your regimen. Don't hesitate to get a personalized exercise program from a qualified fitness consultant.

Natural hormone therapy

Synthetic estrogen has been shown to slow bone loss. However, it does not increase bone density or reverse osteoporosis and it is associated with potentially harmful side effects. If needed, we recommend a safer form of natural estrogen known as tri-estrogen or bi-estrogen.

> Synthetic estrogen has been shown to slow bone loss. However, it does not increase bone density or reverse osteo-porosis and it is asso-ciated with potentially harmful side effects.

Natural progesterone may or may not aid in the prevention and treatment of osteoporosis. More studies need to be done on natural progesterone. However, we often recommend natural progesterone for those seriously at risk or afflicted by osteoporosis. It should be applied 21 days a month if postmenopausal, or the two weeks before menses if not menopausal. Report any vaginal bleeding to your doctor.

Other hormones that may help prevent and/or treat osteoporosis include DHEA and testosterone. Your holistic physician can test for deficiencies of these hormones and recommend individualized treatment. *Note:* DHEA and natural progesterone cream are not sold over the counter in Canada. They are only available through a physician's prescription.

Maximizing joint health

After 50 the risk of osteoporosis increases. Along with bone loss, almost 80% of North Americans also experience some degree of osteoarthritis, a degenerative joint disease in which the cartilage lining the joints wears down. Most affected by osteoarthritis are the weight-bearing joints, such as the hips, knees, and spine, resulting in stiffness, tissue swelling, restricted mobility, and pain. Aspirin and other nonsteroidal anti-inflammatory medications (NSAIDs), such as ibuprofen, are used to reduce joint pain. Although short-term use is usually not harmful, long-term NSAID use can cause digestive upset, ulcers, ringing in the ears, liver and kidney damage. In fact NSAIDS accelerate cartilage destruction and interfere with cartilage synthesis.

Superiority of natural therapies

Natural therapies are the safest and most effective approach for preventing and treating osteoarthritis. Currently, most nutritional-oriented physicians recommend glucosamine and chondroitin sulfate, with excellent results. Glucosamine stimulates the formation of cartilage. It is the thought that as we age, we lose the ability to manufacture glucosamine. The ability of cartilage to regenerate and hold moisture is restricted without glucosamine production.

Several well-designed, double-blind studies have been conducted on glucosamine sulfate. One study involved 252 patients with osteoarthritis of the knee. They were given 500 mg of glucosamine sulfate or a placebo, three times a day for four weeks. The glucosamine group had a significantly greater improvement in pain and mobility over the placebo group.

Glucosamine is often used in combination with chondroitin sulfate, derived from bovine cartilage. It may help repair cartilage tissue in the same way that glucosamine does. Although healthcare professionals debate about the absorption and effectiveness of chondroitin sulfate, we have seen good results with glucosamine when supplemented by itself. We have also had patients who never responded to glucosamine but noticed a dramatic improvement when they took the combination of glucosamine and chondroitin. The adult dosage for either form is 500 mg three times daily.

Antioxidants, found in abundance in fruits and vegetables, also protect against premature degeneration of the joints. Studies show that people with high levels of antioxidants in their diet have a much slower rate of joint deterioration. These antioxidants include vitamins A, C, E, selenium, zinc, beta-carotene, as well as phytochemicals found in plants. A complete multivitamin/mineral formula provides a foundation of these antioxidants.

The omega-3 fatty acids found in fish oils, such as salmon oil, have been shown to reduce the inflammation of osteoarthritis. Consume fish two to three times weekly. If you prefer a fish oil supplement, take 2,000 to 3,000 mg daily.

It's never too late to build strong bones

Ideally, bone health begins when we're young. However, it is never too late to halt or even reverse bone loss. Achieving healthy bones takes a comprehensive strategy that includes proper diet, regular exercise and discontinuing smoking. High-quality supplements should be taken consistently. Start today and optimize your bone health no matter what your age.

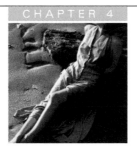

CHAPTER 4

Healthy Breasts, Naturally

There's hardly a woman alive who doesn't feel a chill when she hears the words 'breast cancer.' Now this really is a disease to be reckoned with. Although billions of dollars have been spent on research, the odds of developing breast cancer is increasing, not decreasing. In 1960, one in twenty women developed breast cancer; in 1974, that rose to one in seventeen; still higher in 1994, where one in nine women developed breast cancer.

Whether or not we will get breast cancer can depend more on our diet and lifestyle than on our genes. And even though breast cancer rates are rising among North American women (and men) there are exciting nutritional breakthroughs based on good science that can help us prevent this terrifying disease.

Breast cancer—Let's beat the odds

Isn't it curious that the common factors that prevent PMS, Menopausal symptoms, and encourage healthy bones can also help us avoid breast cancer? More than 200 epidemiological studies indicate that a diet high in fruits and vegetables lead to a decrease in cancer and that 35% of all cancers are directly linked to diet and nutrition. Only a small percentage of breast cancers are strongly genetic in nature, somewhere between 5-10%. Therefore, diet, nutritional deficiencies, lifestyle, stress, environmental toxins, and hormonal factors must be addressed to prevent and treat this disease.

> Isn't it curious that the common factors that prevent PMS, Menopausal symptoms, and encourage healthy bones can also help us avoid breast cancer?

Eat a high-fiber, plant-based diet that includes lots of vegetables, fruits, grains, legumes, herbs, nuts, and seeds. Try to eat organic whenever possible. Avoid the saturated fats found in red meat, luncheon meats and high-fat dairy products. Consume foods containing glucaric acid (apples, carrots, spinach, oranges, grapefruit, cherries, broccoli). Keep alcohol intake to a minimum and engage in a regular exercise program.

And of course, quit smoking. Just these few changes in diet and lifestyle can reduce your risk of ever getting breast cancer. But the news gets better:

Calcium D-Glucarate—a cutting-edge detoxifier

One way to prevent breast cancer from ever developing is to harness the body's own detoxifying systems. A complex system called Phase II detoxification works by conjugating (binding) dangerous toxins (including carcinogens and excess estrogens) to water soluble substances, allowing them to quickly pass through the body and excreted. According to noted cancer scientist Dr. Thomas Slaga "One of the most important Phase II reactions in our body is the conjugation reactions that use D-glucarate. D-glucarate helps the body remove carcinogens, toxins, and compounds that are no longer needed." Not only does D-glucarate help to render toxins harmless in the liver, it also prevents this process from being reversed. An enzyme called beta-glucuronidase can change the harmless molecule back into a harmful toxin before it can be excreted. A related compound called D-glucaro-1,4-lactone (GL), inhibits the activity of beta-glucuronidase, allowing the toxins to be eliminated. Dr. Slaga comments on the value of oral

> "Oral ingestion of calcium D-glucarate has been shown to inhibit beta-glucuronidase. This means the body is better able to get rid of carcinogens and waste products."
>
> Dr. Thomas Slaga

Calcium-D-glucarate: "Oral ingestion of calcium D-glucarate has been shown to inhibit beta-glucuronidase. This means the body is better able to get rid of carcinogens and waste products. In one animal study, a single dose of calcium D-glucarate inhibited beta-glucuronidase activity by 57 percent in the blood, 44 percent in the liver, 39 percent in the intestines and 37 percent in the lungs. In the same study, beta-glucuronidase activity in the microflora was inhibited by 70 percent in the small intestine and by 54 percent in the colon. Calcium D-glucarate has the greatest potential as a compound against carcinogens for a number of reasons: (1) It is non-toxic when orally administered; (2) it is converted to the active GL form in the body, which inhibits beta-glucuronidase; and (3) it provides for the slow release of GL after ingestion."

What do the studies show?

Although human studies on Calcium D-glucarate are just beginning, animal studies show that it can inhibit breast, colon, lung, liver, skin and urinary bladder cancers.

Excess circulating estrogens are also implicated in breast cancer. D-glucarate reduced estrogen and pro-gesterone receptor levels in rats that had chemically-induced breast cancers.

For more information please read ***D-Glucarate: A Nutrient Against Cancer*** by Thomas Slaga, Ph. D.

Rosemary—an aromatic herb to be reckoned with

More than just a pretty bush or an aromatic herb for roast lamb, rosemary contains potent antioxidants and other compounds that can prevent or block cancer formation. In one study, rats with a likelihood of developing mammary tumors were given rosemary extract. The rosemary extract resulted in a 47 percent decrease in mammary tumor formation compared to controls. Rats given rosemary (as one percent of their diet) two weeks prior to tumor-causing DMBA administration had 76 percent less of the carcinogen bind to their DNA than the rats fed a control diet. Tissue culture experiments on human liver and bronchial cells show that rosemary extract provides dual protection: It may increase liver enzymes that deactivate carcinogens and reduce the enzymes that enhance carcinogen formation. Take advantage of the cancer-fighting properties of this remarkable aromatic herb and use it liberally.

The extraordinary cruciferous family—Indole-3-carbinol and sulforaphane

Broccoli, cauliflower, cabbage, Brussels sprouts, kale— these vegetables are loaded with indoles and sulforaphane, powerful cancer-fighting chemicals. Indoles activate detoxification enzymes in the intestinal tract, bind to chemical carcinogens, rendering them inactive, and improve estrogen balance, reducing the risk of breast cancer. Indole 3 carbinol helps in the breakdown of estrogen into "good" metabolites and less of the "bad" metabolites of estrogen.

Animal studies show that sulforaphane (a naturally occurring isothiocyanate) is also an effective cancer fighter. In particular sulforaphane helps with Phase II detoxification (Calcium D-glucarate also enhances this detoxification process). These enzymes neutralize dangerous carcinogens before they can damage DNA and promote cancer.

Silymarin—the active ingredient in Milk Thistle

World-renowned ethnobotanist, Dr. James Duke, can't say enough good about milk thistle: "This is my favorite liver protector. The liver processes drugs and environmental toxins, so it's under constant assault. Anyone who drinks alcohol, takes drugs...or comes in contact with any pollutants might benefit from this herb."

We would like to add that anyone trying to enhance breast health and prevent cancer should also know about this herb. The active ingredients in milk thistle are flavonoids comprised of silybin, silydianin and silychristin—collectively known as silymarin. Researchers are giving these flavonoids rave reviews for their ability to support liver function. As mentioned earlier in this book, a healthy liver improves our estrogen balance by metabolizing estrogen properly. The silymarin component is a powerful antioxidant and free radical scavenger and it also helps to increase glutathione, an antioxidant that can detoxify a wide range of hormones, drugs and toxins.

Reduce your risk—a preventive formula based on research

Based on cutting-edge research into the cancer-protective effects of select phytochemicals, Dr. Mark and I have designed a formula for women of all ages who want to optimize their breast health and reduce their risk of breast cancer. Each ingredient of the breast formula contributes an important component to total breast health. The protective phytochemicals in the formula are standardized extracts, ensuring consistency and potency. Unlike isolated pharmaceuticals, these extracts are found in the base of the whole plant. While we're not suggesting that you don't have to eat your broccoli, this formulation might be ideal for women who can't or won't eat copious amounts of cruciferous vegetables everyday.

> Only a small percentage of breast cancers are strongly genetic in nature, somewhere between 5-10%. Therefore, diet, nutritional deficiencies, lifestyle, stress, environmental toxins, and hormonal factors must be addressed to prevent and treat this disease.

I recommend the following Breast Health formula by Natural Factors® for the prevention of breast cancer, and as part of a comprehensive protocol for the treatment of breast cancer. It is also indicated for fibrocystic breast syndrome and for women currently on hormone replacement.

> Calcium D-Glucarate ....135 mg
> Rosemary Extract ....15 mg
> Indole-3-carbinol ....50 mg
> Sulforaphane ....70 mg
> Silymarin ....35 mg

Dosage: Take 3 capsules daily or as directed by your healthcare practitioner.

Cancer and Cardiovascular protection with soy

Soy deserves special mention because of its well-researched hormone balancing and cancer preventing properties. In addition to reducing symptoms such as hot flashes, soy contains powerful anticancer phytochemicals. Asian populations (who consume large amounts of soybeans) have lower rates of breast, colon, and prostate cancer. A review of 81 articles related to phytoestrogens, soy products, and diets with high phytoestrogen content, concluded that phytoestrogens are among the dietary factors that protect against cancer and heart disease in vegetarians. The phytoestrogens in soy can block estrogen receptors in certain hormone-dependent tissues such as the breast and uterus. The two most important soy phytoestrogens appear to be the isoflavones, genistein and daidzein. In the body, they are converted to phytoestrogens, positively affecting hormone metabolism and estrogen activity. Specifically, genistein reduces the risk of estrogen-sensitive tumor growth. Women who consume a traditional Japanese diet excrete 1,000 times more genistein than those from societies with high breast cancer rates.

Soy also contains phytochemicals that benefit the heart and arteries. These include saponins, phytosterols, and isoflavones. Soy has been shown in many studies to lower levels of LDL cholesterol and triglycerides. Consuming one to two ounces of soy protein for an average of four weeks can lower abnormally high total and LDL (harmful) cholesterol by 10 to 20 percent. Studies have also shown that soy increases HDL (good) cholesterol.

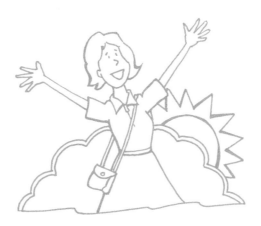

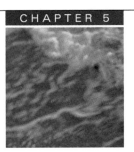

CHAPTER 5

Pulling it all Together

Y ou are in charge of your health. It is important to live a healthy lifestyle not only to prevent PMS, to ease menopause or prevent cancer, but also to ensure that you have a quality of life that is well worth living. You can feel more energetic and healthier overall by following the recommendations in this book. If you find your symptoms intolerable even with these powerful natural remedies get a full complement of tests done by a natural health professional to give you additional guidance. Hormone balance, along with a good diet, nutritional supplements and exercise, can make a huge difference in your health and well-being. I hope you will follow these natural ways to being a healthy woman.

Yours in good health,

Angela Stengler ND

Dr. Angela Stengler ND

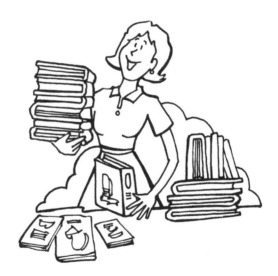

PMS Case Studies

Tina (37 years old) came to me wanting a treatment for her horrible PMS. Her husband came as well, explaining to me that she was terribly irritable, emotional and very hard to live with the weeks preceding her period. After talking with Tina I took note of the fact that she owned her own business, was very committed to her work, did not eat regular meals and had a teenage son at home who was causing her some distress. She told me that she could not spend a lot of time changing her lifestyle and did not have time to cook.

I made some simple dietary changes for Tina to follow and I had her start the Natural Factors® PMS formula. After her next period, her *neighbour* called me up telling me what a different person she was and he wanted me to send her more of the PMS formula to his house so she would for sure get it!!! It has been three months since I last saw her and she continues to do well on the formula and will probably lessen the dosage within the next two months.

Renee was a young 27 year old woman suffering from mood swings, horrible breast tenderness and bloating two weeks prior to her menstrual cycle. She was willing to make some dietary changes and take supplements so I suggested a whole foods diet, extra vitamin E and the Natural Factors® PMS formula. She noticed some improvement after taking the formula for one cycle but she showed dramatic improvement after taking the formula for two cycles. She continued to use the formula for a total of 5 months and now uses it as needed the last two weeks of her cycle. She mentioned to me that using the formula made her feel so much better that it was easy to change her lifestyle which has enabled her to lose 10 pounds, feel more energetic and much more healthy.

MENOPAUSE Case Studies:

Elizabeth is a 47 year old mother of two with the beginning symptoms of menopause. She was experiencing horrible mood swings, hot flashes and irregular periods. I prescribed the Menopause Formula by Natural Factors®. Her daily hot flashes went away after three weeks but she was still experiencing night sweats. I suggested she double the dose of the menopause formula (4 capsules a day) and add soy isoflavones to her regimen before bed. Now she can sleep through the night without waking up in a sweat. This formula helped her so much she felt enough energy to start an exercise program and follow a plant based diet. She is basically sailing through menopause!

Karen is a 57 year old women on synthetic hormone replacement for 7 years. She came to me because her menopausal symptoms have gotten worse not better while on this medication. She could not sleep, had terrible mood swings, and had a very low sex drive. Since she had her ovaries and uterus, and did not have any risk factors for osteoporosis, I had her start the Natural Factors® Menopause Formula (she was still on the synthetic hormone replacement) as directed on the bottle. After two weeks she could not believe how well she felt. After two more weeks she gradually stopped the synthetic hormone replacement therapy. She continues to do well on the Menopause Formula and has started an exercise/fitness program and is taking cooking classes.

"Helping people enjoy optimum health is my goal. Check out our website and let us know your experiences."

Dr. Angela Stengler

www.thenaturalphysician.com

References

Long, J, Rybacki J: *The Essential Guide to Prescription Drugs.*
   pp. 979-985. New York: Harper Perennial, 1995.
Weiss, RF: *Herbal Medicine*, p. 317.
   Sweden: Beaconsfield Publishers Ltd. 1988.
Amann, W: *Removing and obstipation using agnolyt.*
   Ther Gegenw 104:1263-1265, 1965.
Peteres-Welter B. Albrecht M: *Menstrual abnormalities and PMS.*
   Vitex Agnus-castus in a study of application.
   Therapiewoche Gynakol 7:49-52, 1994.
Dittmar F W, et al: *Premenstrual syndrome: treatment with a*
   phytopharmaceutical. Therapiewoche Gynakol 5(1):60-8, 1992.
Peteres-Welter B. Albrecht M: *Menstrual abnormalities and PMS.*
   Vitex Agnus-castus in a study of application.
   Therapiewoche Gynakol 7:49-52, 1994.
Milewicz, A. et al: *Vitex Agnus-castus extract in the treatment of*
   luteal phase defects due to latent hyperprolactinemia: results
   of a randomized, placebo-controlled, double-blind study.
   Arzneim Forsch Drug Res 43(7): 752-6, 1993.
Hobbs, C: *Taraxacum officinale: A monograph and literature review.*
   In: Eclectic Dispensatory.
   Portland: Eclectic Medical Pubications, 1989.
Mowrey, D: *Herbal Tonic Therapies.* p. 164.
   New Canaan: Keats Publishing, Inc., 1993.
Gladstar R: *Herbal Healing for Women*, p. 240.
   New York. Simon and Schuster. 1993.
Goldin BR et al: *Estrogen patterns and plasma levels in vegetarian*
   and omnivorous women. New Engl J Med 307:1542-7, 1982.
Werbach, MR: *Nutritional Influences on Illness.* 2nd Edition.
   Pp. 540-541 (review). Tarzana: Third Line Press, 1993.
Jones, DV: *Influence of dietary fat on self-reported menstrual symptoms.*
   Physiol Behav 40(4): 438-87, 1987.
Rossignol AM et al:*Prevalence and severity of the premenstrual syndrome:*
   effects of foods and beverages that are sweet or high in sugar
   content. J Reprod Med 36(2): 131-6, 1991.
Barr, W: *Pyridoxine supplements in the premenstrual syndrome.*
   The Practitioner 228:425-427, 1984.

Thys-Jacobs S, Starkey P, Bernstein D, Tian J , Amer J Obstet Gynecol 1998 August:179(2):444-52, *Calcium carbonate and the premenstrual syndrome: effects on premenstrual and menstrual symptoms. Premenstrual Syndrome Study Group.*

Sherwood, RA et al: *Magnesium and the premenstrual syndrome.* Ann Clin Biochem 23:667-70, 1986.

Judd AM et al: *Zinc and copper levels in premenstrual syndrome.* Fertility & Sterility 62:313-20, 1994.

Horrobin DF: *The role of essential fatty acids and prostaglandins in the premenstrual syndrome.* J Reprod Med 28: 465-68, 1993.

London RS et al: *The effect of alpha-tocopherol on premenstrual symptomatology: a double-blind study, 11, endocrine correlates.* J Am Col Nutr 3: 351-356, 1984.

Brayshaw ND et al: *Thyroid hypofunction in premenstrual syndrome.* New Engl J Med 315: 1486-7, 1986.

Wright, Jonathan and John Morgenthaler: *The many functions of a horse. Natural Hormone Replacement for Women Over 45,* p 25 Petaluma: Smart Publications, 1998.

Physicians' Desk Reference. 52nd Edition. Montvale: Medical Economics Company, Inc., 1998.

Rose DP: *Dietary fiber, phytoestrogens, and breast cancer.* Nutrition 8:47-51, 1992.

Duker EM, Kopanski L, Jarry H, Wuttke W.: *Effects of extracts from Cimicifuga racemosa on gonadotropin release in menopausal women and ovariectomized rats.* Planta Medica 57:420-24. 1991.

Stolze H: *The other way to treat symptoms of menopause.* Gyne 1:14-16, 1982.

Harnischfeger G, Stolze H: *Black Cohosh.* Notabene Medici 10:446-50, 1980.

Peteres-Welter C, Albrecht M: *Menstrual abnormalities and PMS: Vitex agnus-castus in a study of application.* Therapiewoche Gynakol 7:49-52, 1994.

Gladstar, Rosemary: *Herbal Healing For Women.* pg. 244. New York: Fireside Books. 1993.

Moscarini, M, et al: *New perspectives in the treatment of postmenopausal osteoporosis: ipriflavone. Gynecol. Endrocrinol* 8 (3):203-207, 1994.

Reid, IR, et al: *Effects of calcium supplementation on bone loss in postmenopausal women.* New Engl J Med 13:S11-16, 1993.

Smith EL, et al: *Calcium supplementation and bone loss in middle-aged women.* Am J Clin Nutr 50:833-842, 1989.

Abraham, GE: *The importance of magnesium in the management of primary postmenopausal osteoporosis.* J Nutr Med 2, 1991.

Ooms, ME, et al: *Prevention of bone loss by vitamin D supplementation in elderly women: a randomized double-blind study.*
J Clin Endocrinol Metabol 80:1052-58, 1995.

Chapu, MC, et al: *Effects of calcium and cholecalciferol treatment for three years on hip fractures in elderly women.*
BMJ 308: 1081-82, 1992.

Hyams, et al: *Scurvy, megaloblastic anemia and osteoporosis.*
Br J Clin Pract 117:332-40, 1963.

Wolf, SL, et al: *Reducing frailty and falls in older persons: an investigation of tai chi and computerized balance training.*
J Amer Geri Soc 44: 489-97, 1996.

Shield MJ: *Anti-inflammatory drugs and their effects on cartilage synthesis and renal function.*
Eur J Rheumatoid Inflam 13:7-17, 1993.

Brooks PM, et al: *NSAID and osteoarthritis: help or hindrance.*
J Rheumatol 9:3-5, 1982.

Noack W, et al: *Glucosamine sulfate in osteoarthritis of the knee.*
Osteoarthritis Cartilage 2:51-9, 1994.

Slaga, Thomas J. M.D.: *D-Glucarate: a nutrient against cancer.*
Keats Publishing. 1999.

Dwivedi, C. et al.: *Effect of calcium glucarate on beta-glucuronidase activity and glucarate content of certain vegetables and fruits.*
Biochem Med and Met Biol. 43(2):83-92, 1990.

Slaga, Thomas J. M.D.: *D-Glucarate: a nutrient against cancer.*
Keats Publishing. 1999.

Walaszek, Z. et al: *Effect of dietary glucarate on estrogen receptors and growth of 7, 12-dimethylbenz(a)anthracene-induced rat mammary carcinomas.* Breast Cancer Res. Treat. 12, 128. 1988.

Singletary, K.W. et al.: *Inhibition of 7,12-dimethylbenz(a)anthracene (DMBA)-induced mammary tumorigenesis and of in vivo formation of mammary DMBA-DNA adducts by rosemary extract.*
Cancer Lett. Nov. 60(2):169-75, 1991.

Amagase, H. et al.: *Dietary rosemary suppresses 7,12-dimethylbenz-(a)anthracene binding to rat mammary cell DNA.*
J. Nutr. 126:1475-80, 1996.

Offord, E.A. et al.: *Mechanisms involved in the chemoprotective effects of rosemary extract studied in human liver and bronchial cells.* Cancer Lett. 114:275-81, 1997.

Zeligs, M.: *Diet and estrogen: the crucifer connection.* J. of Med. Food (2):67-82, 1998.

Duke, James A. Ph.D.: *The Green Pharmacy: New Discoveries in Herbal Remedies for Common Diseases and Conditions from the World's Foremost Authority on Healing Herbs.* Rodale Press. 1997.